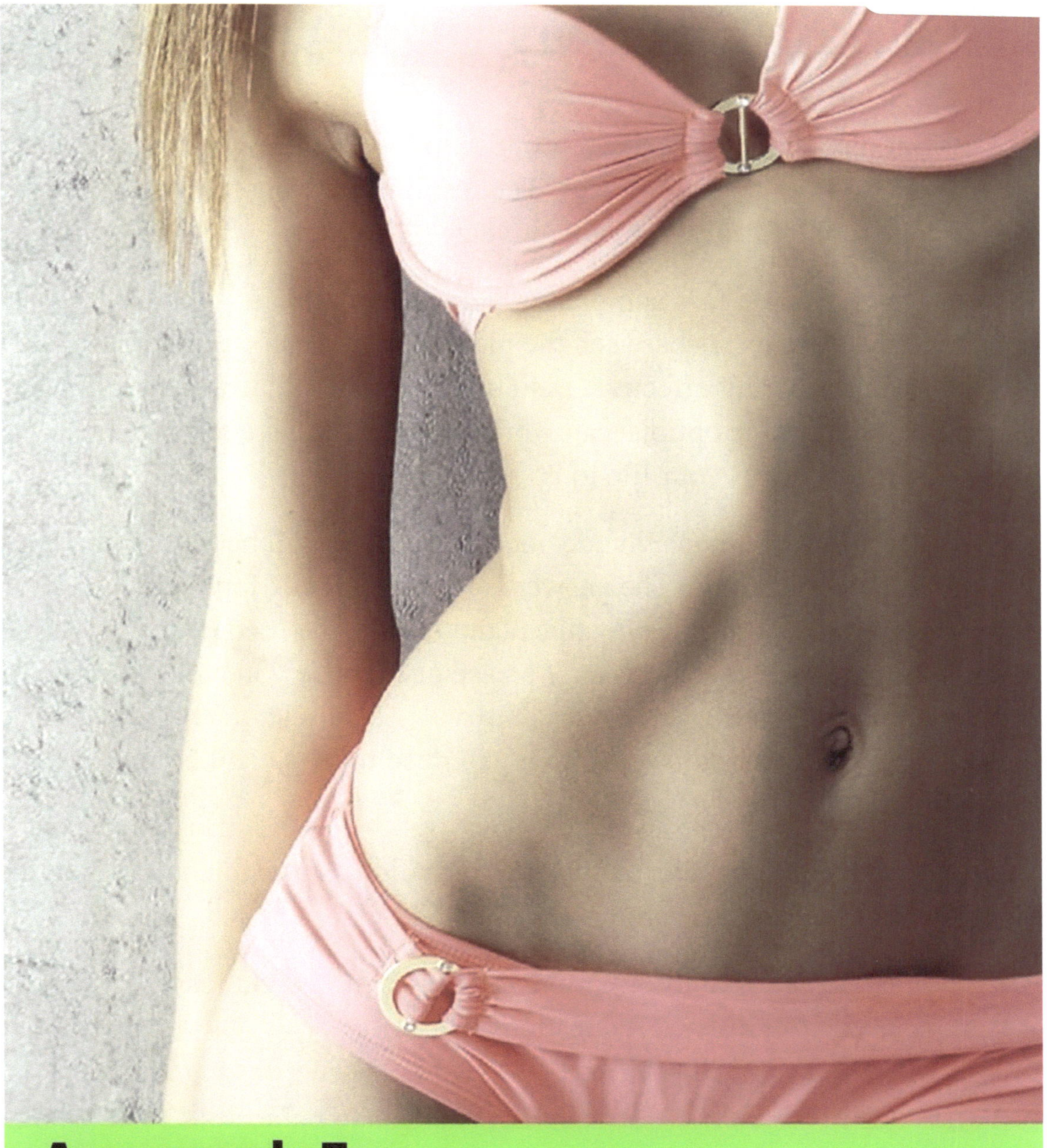

Approach For
Natural Weight Loss Plan

Kelley O'Hara

A Sensible Approach For Natural Weight Loss Plan

Every year millions of people make a promise to lose weight, yet most of those people struggle to keep those promises. The result is the weight stays on and more damage is done to their health for another year.

There are so many weight loss and dieting options available it is almost impossible to understand the differences between the plans. If that wasn't enough, how do you know which plans are truly effective. If so many people fail at weight loss what works? In theory all of the options can work but you will have to make huge changes in every aspect of your life to be successful.

Whatever weight loss approach you decide to take there will be work to be done and obstacles to be overcome. The answer is really the same for everyone; you need to change the amount of food you eat and change the foods you eat. When you couple those two changes with an increase in exercise you will lose weight. Exercise is important so that you have a daily calorie deficiency. A daily calorie deficiency, what in the world is that? You will need to be patient because I will explain that later.

In this article I have put together as much information as possible given that this is an article and not a novel. So here we go:

I've tried to include as much information as I can about weight loss, so you won't leave this book with too many left questions to ask.

Let's Get Started!

In the morning when you get dressed are you frustrated with the image you see in the mirror? What's happened to your body, your tummy is getting flabby, your waist is getting wider and your hips are getting heavier. If that wasn't enough you look at your face and see a few wrinkles starting and a little extra jiggle under your chin.

What can you do to stop this from getting worse and what is happening to your body when you gain weight. These are the questions that I will answer in this article. I will show you how to lose weight and keep it off.

It is a national 'sport' to 'people watch' at the beach. But when you do this you find yourself comparing your body to every slim, tanned and toned body you see. It is a cruel fact of nature that there are some people who never have to watch what they eat, who don't have to exercise much, and who just are blessed with a metabolism that burns fast. These people never think about how much they are eating, when they are eating, or how many calories they are consuming.

We place so much importance on our weight, why is our weight so important? The simple truth is two reasons - how we look and how we feel.

Physical Appearance

If people are honest they will tell you that they don't want to be fat. In our society our appearance is a determining factor as to how we will be accepted by others, which opportunities we will be offered and, most importantly, our self-esteem. Self-esteem is a powerful force in our lives and it plays out in every aspect of our day. If you believe that your body is not desirable then you can become depressed, sad, and even develop depression. This depression or sadness can lead to the development of binge or emotional eating. If that happens you enter a vicious cycle of being depressed, eating to feel a sense of emotional contentment then getting more depressed because of what you ate.

Doctors have been documenting the emotional toll of being obese. It has been established that a person's sense of self-worth and emotional stability can be destroyed when becoming obese. The emotional consequences of being obese over a long period of time can be crushing and may require intense therapy from a primary care physician and therapist.

Take a second to answer these questions, be honest so that the answers will help you.

- Have you ever looked in the mirror and thought you looked ugly?
- Are you comfortable with the body you see in the mirror?
- Are you worried about your partner's opinion of your body?
- Do you find yourself thinking about what other people think about you when they look at you?

If you answered 'yes' to any of those questions then it is very possible that your weight is affecting how you perceive yourself and how you believe others may perceive you. Life is very difficult when your physical appearance can exert such a powerful influence. So, you have two choices:

1) Change

2) Live with it

If you picked #2 then you must also be prepared to live with the emotional consequences of being overweight.

It is my hope that you chose the first option, that you want to change and in another section of the article I will lay the ground work for you to do just that.

Health Concerns

Most likely you are aware of the numerous problems to your health if you are obese. If you are 20 lbs. overweight you can really begin to experience the ill effects of being overweight.

The problems from being overweight can present themselves in many ways. That nagging lower back pain is it from last night's pick-up basketball game or is your back sore because your body is struggling to function with that additional 20 lbs. Twenty pounds might not sound like much but grab four 5 lb. bags of potatoes and

carry them around for a few hours. I think at the end of that experiment you will have a much greater appreciation for what your body has to deal with when you gain weight.

When your weight reaches a certain level, when you pass being overweight and become obese, you put enormous strain on all the parts of your body such as your heart, your joints, your feet, your lungs.

Once you are overweight, you set yourself up for life threatening health problems and diseases. You are now a candidate for the FATAL FOUR......stroke, heart attack, high blood pressure, and diabetes. I'm sure you don't want any of those in your life, so commit right now that you will make the changes you need to make to live a healthier and longer life.

Medical Fact:

In one study a group of people, 5881 to be exact, were monitored over a 14-year period. The doctors were looking for a link between people being overweight and heart failure. What the doctors discovered was if a person is just 'overweight', not obese that person will have a 34% greater chance of experiencing heart failure.

The report was even more startling for an obese person. For those people who were categorized as obese the risk of heart failure jumped to 104% versus someone whose weight was in the 'normal' range.

Did that get your attention? I hope so.

Overweight Versus Obese

I have been using the terms 'overweight' and 'obese' but I have not defined either term. To clarify exactly the difference between the two here are the definitions I will use:

Obese: doctors consider you obese if you are 20 to 30 percent over your 'ideal' body weight

Overweight: doctors consider you overweight if your body mass index (BMI) is 25 or over. (Just to give you a point of reference that would mean you were 5 to 15 percent over your ideal body weight. OUCH!!)

If you would like to find out what your 'ideal' weight is here is a link that you will find helpful:

http://www.halls.md/ideal-weight/body.htm

Never lose sight of the fact that you are at a much higher risk of experiencing the FATAL FOUR if you are just overweight. That fact alone should convince you want to make the changes in your life to avoid that type of misery.

It is now time to take control of your life, to make the changes that allow you to live a longer and healthier life.

Why We Gain Weight

There are endless reasons why people gain weight. The reasons can range from simply overeating and not getting enough exercise to burn off the calories from the food to as complicated as being passed from one generation to the next genetically.

To have a true understanding of how a person will lose weight, you first have to understand why you gain weight. Next I am going to describe some of the reasons why people gain weight.

Calories We Consume: Don't Eat More Than You Can Burn

The simplest reason why we gain weight is that we consume more food, giving us more calories, than we can use in one day. Anytime you eat anything your body converts the food into sugars. This is something our bodies have learned to do over the millions of years the human species has existed. Your body knows that it must store excess 'energy' so if food is scarce the body can keep functioning. If, for some reason, food is no longer available the body draws upon the resources of sugar to provide fuel for our bodies. This meant that if a human had to continue to hunt and forage for food their body would be able to perform everything they asked of it.

The advantage our predecessors had over us is that they had to work very hard to find food so that excess fat was burned off very rapidly. That meant that they didn't experience the same problems with obesity that we do

Today, for most of us, food is readily available, so we can over eat and indulge ourselves. This means that now we must find ways to burn off the extra calories to allow us to maintain our weight. When we understand how the body stores and burns fat we then have the tools to understand how not to gain weight. Our society and our standard of living has made it too easy to eat too much, too often.

4 Reasons For Weight Gain:

(1) Low Metabolism

Whether you have a slow, normal or fast metabolism can be attributed partly to genetics. However we can increase our metabolism by taking some simple steps.

When you can't remember why you exercise just think about this, muscles burn fat and they continue to burn fat after you have finished your exercise. That's right our muscles are like having a fat burning furnace inside our bodies. When you sit all night in front of the TV or computer your muscles are not burning any fat which also means that your body isn't burning any calories. The result is that the calories our muscles should be burning, but aren't because we are sitting around, are now turned into fat by our bodies. This is exactly what we don't want.

If you exercise the following occurs:

- You build and/or tone your muscles.
- The muscles in your body need fuel so they burn the stored fat.
- As you exercise you raise your heart rate which is beneficial to your entire body.
- You finish your exercise but your muscles continue to require fuel so they continue to burn the stored fat. When you are active your entire body benefits, heart, lungs, muscles, joints, and mind, and all this will increase your metabolism which makes it easier for you to lose weight.

To Increase Your Metabolism:

- **Start out with an exercise routine that lasts 20 minutes** and repeat the routine 3 times a week. This will begin to raise your metabolism and get you on the right path to lose weight.

- **Portion control**. We have developed a distorted concept of the amount of food that we should consume at each meal. To make it easy always think smaller. Begin to plan for 5-6 small meals a day. The plan would include a healthy breakfast, then a small healthy snack, lunch, another small snack and then a healthy dinner. The healthy snacks will keep your metabolism at a good rate and will also prevent you from having a craving to go get something sweet and unhealthy.

- **EAT!!!!** Never starve yourself because you will force your body to go into 'starvation mode'. We spoke briefly about this but it bears repeating, if your body senses that it is not receiving adequate nourishment it will begin to store fat. This is a recipe for disaster if you are trying to lose weight. Your body will win and the pounds will not come off.

- **Walk**. At every opportunity find a reason to walk. It can be as simple as parking your car far away from the building you work in so your walk is long or you can walk up the stairs instead of taking the elevator. Be creative and find opportunities to walk. If you can schedule the time a 30 minute walk at least three times a week will work wonders for your health and metabolism.

- **Never and I mean NEVER skip breakfast**. Your body has been resting and repairing for the last 8 hours and now it needs fuel to get you going for the day. Take the time to plan a healthy breakfast and don't settle for the easy route of grabbing a donut or other pastry.

- **Understand your eating habits**. How and what you eat will determine, to a large extent, your ability to lose weight. Do you sit down for a huge dinner loaded with carbs, fats and sweets? At meal time do you have a smaller portion of lean meats, veggies and carbs? Do you take your time enjoying your meal or do you eat as fast as you can? Examine your patterns of eating and see which patterns you can alter the easiest and then begin making the necessary changes.

(2) How You Eat

- What does a typical meal look like? Is your plate filled with fatty foods that are high in calories? These foods are difficult for your body to utilize and you put yourself at a greater risk of the FATAL FOUR if this type of food is on you plate. Examples would be deep fried foods, fast food French fries, rich creamy sauces.

- Are you a fast eater? The rate at which you eat your dinner is important. If you eat too fast your brain does not get the signal that you are full until you have over eaten. The easiest method to slow yourself down at a meal is to put your fork down between bites. Take the time to taste your food and enjoy what you are eating before you pick up your fork for more.

- When you take your time to chew your food that allows the saliva in your mouth longer to break down the food. Give your body every chance it has to break down the food and extract all the nutrients it can.

- Portion size: Eat smaller but more often. We discussed this earlier; you can increase your metabolism by giving it a constant source of fuel to break down. It is also easier on your stomach and digestive system to have smaller amounts of food to break down. Be nice to your body and it will pay you huge dividends.

(3) Genetics

What you family has given you to work with: It is true that genetics play a role in a person's ability to gain or lose weight but genetics are not the entire story. By taking the right approach you can make sure your body is nourished and healthy and not gain weight despite what your parents and grandparents look like. Your genetics play a role in determining your metabolism and your tendency to gain weight but do not let this stop you from taking the steps you need to live as healthy a life as possible. Remember, this is your life so you are responsible for taking care of yourself.

Exercise

Yes it is true, we all need to exercise. Nothing is as beneficial as getting your heart going and toning your muscles. The benefits of exercise touch all parts of your body and life so make sure to schedule time for a workout. I know that life is hectic but all you need to do is 20 minutes three times a week to begin to help your body. Remember, you don't need to run a marathon or climb Mt. Everest, all you need to do is elevate your heart rate and keep it elevated for 20 minutes. Start out easy and work up to more strenuous activates. Never over exert and never begin any exercise program without checking with your doctor.

Let's just summarize the benefits of exercise:

- **You will feel great**: That alone should be enough to get all of us out and exercising. Isn't that a good start? Exercise changes you inside and out, nothing else has such a dramatic systemic effect.
- **Muscles:** Exercise builds and tones your muscles. As a result your metabolism is increased which makes it easier to lose weight. The more muscles you have working for you the more fat you will burn.
- **Stress:** Exercise is great for lowering the stress levels in your life and in your body. According to many studies not only will exercising for 20 minutes three times week be beneficial for your metabolism but it will also lower your stress levels.
- **Calories burned:** Exercise demolishes calories. Later in this article I will discuss the process of successful long term weight loss and at that point you will have a better understanding of the importance of burning calories. The simple concept is when you burn more calories than you eat you lose weight.

Always remember that exercise is any physical activity, you can walk, ride a bike, swim, or anything that gets you moving. Don't get hung up on not being able to do a lot at the start. The most important thing is to start and stick with it.

Not exercising is a guarantee to gaining weight. If you continue to eat as usual and continue the 'couch potato' mentality then you are setting yourself up for a difficult life of illness and disease.

Who Is To Blame: Society, You or McDonalds?

There are many people who blame the rapidly rising obesity rate in the U.S. on the fast food industry. They believe that the option to 'super-size', eat deep fried French fries and a host of other fat rich, empty calorie foods should take the blame. They say that our lifestyle of rushing everywhere and doing six things at once does not allow us to prepare healthy meals for us and our families

But is that the whole truth? I don't think so. Everyone has a choice. In many cases it comes down to access to the proper foods or knowledge of how to prepare healthy meals but given the choice I believe that most people would want to live a healthy life.

We have the opportunity today to make that choice. We live in a world where we can access information on any subject. So let's start today to make the right choices, take the time to plan and prepare healthy meals and leave the bad habits from the past in the past.

Good Nutrition

To lose weight you must do two things, practice good nutrition and make time to exercise. Without the proper nutrition your chances of experiencing successful long term weight loss is dramatically reduced. Let's make sure we understand one fact, crash diets do not qualify as proper nutrition.

Proper nutrition means you are consuming healthy, balanced, and well-rounded meals. It means you are practicing portion control, understanding how many calories you need to eat to experience weight loss and still be healthy, and limiting your intake of sweets. Current wisdom says that if you can create a daily 500 calorie deficit you will lose weight. That calorie deficit is achieved by exercise and meal planning. If you do this you can lose approximately one pound a week. One pound a week may seem inadequate but think of what you are doing. You are making huge changes in your life; you are changing what you eat, when you eat, and how you eat. That is a lot to undertake and losing one pound a week is the type of weight loss that you can sustain over a long period of time. Simply put, if you can lose one pound a week you will lose 52 lbs. in one year. Now that is an incredible accomplishment.

Calorie Intake

The calorie deficit must be subtracted from the total calories you consume each day to maintain your weight. For example, a man eating 2000 calories a day could cut back 250 calories in food intake and step up his workout to burn an extra 250 calories every day. If he follows that for one week he will have created a 3500

calorie deficit for the week and will have lost one pound. (Note: you must burn off 3500 calories to lose 1lb. of fat so you need a daily 500 calorie deficit to maintain your 1lb. per week weight loss.)

Minimum Calorie Intake

Here are a few general 'rules' regarding calorie intake:

Women: should consume at least 1,200 calories a day, or 1,000 less than your maintenance calories (maintenance value = how many calories you need to maintain your current weight). The Harris-Benedict formula is one of the leading ways to calculate your maintenance value.

Men: should consume at least 1,800 calories per day, or 1,000 less than your maintenance calories.

The Harris-Benedict Formula

The Harris Benedict Equation is a formula which will help you determine your BMI. I have provided a link for you to follow so that you can determine your BMI, BMR and the total number of calories you can consume every day. Please check out this resource because it will provide you with valuable information. http://www.bmi-calculator.net/bmr-calculator

I hope you followed the link and determined how many calories you can consume each day. This is an important starting point that will allow you to determine the foods to eat and how much you can eat.

Many people are attracted to crash diets. Crash diets, where you are only consuming 1,000 calories or less per day, are attractive to people because with a crash diet you can lose significant weight over a very short period of time. The problem with crash diets is your body will not function, over the long term, with this limited caloric intake. As a result of the reduced consumption of calories your body will begin to consume the lean muscle mass and as I discussed earlier your muscles play an integral role in the burning of calories. With a crash diet you will lose weight but damage your body in the process. The other problem is that you cannot remain on a crash diet for very long and as soon as you stop the diet you will gain back all the weight and probably add a few pounds.

In summary crash diets do not work and are unhealthy because:

- Starving your body will not provide you with long term weight loss.
- You need your muscles and a crash diet will decrease the amount of lean muscle mass within your body making it even more difficult for you to lose weight in the future.
- Your metabolism needs fuel to operate effectively and when you eat less it will slow down your metabolism. You must provide your body with fuel at regular intervals to allow your metabolism to be at a high level.

Keeping Track of Your Calories

When you begin a weight loss program it is important to know how many calories you are consuming. It is worth the extra effort to write down how many calories you consume and you will find as the process goes along you will develop a sense of how much to eat. It will take a few minutes to write down the calories from the food container but you will provide yourself with the information you need to be successful at weight loss.

Now is the time to get really serious about what you eat. Look at every meal, what is on the table, do you see breads, rolls, high fat salad dressing, and creamy sauces. You need to understand what you can eat, how much you can eat, and how much exercise it will take to burn off what you eat. You now have to take control over food so monitor each meal and make sure that what you put on your plate allows you to reach your daily calorie goal.

As a general rule of thumb, figure that each meal will have between 500 - 1000 calories. Using this as your guide you can plan your meals for the day and know, with confidence, that you will reach but not exceed your goals.

The Food We Eat

In conjunction with the number of calories you eat it is important to also pay close attention to the types of food you eat. Quite simply put, 100 grams of carrots has far less fat than 100 grams of pastry.

We have many choices regarding the types of food we eat. There is high fat, high calorie, processed, and organic foods to name just a few. Each type of food will affect your ability to lose weight so be intelligent about the foods you choose. I am not saying that you cannot have foods from all the groups but I am saying that you must limit your intake of foods that are high in fat if you are serious about losing weight.

High-Fat Foods

It is common knowledge that high fat foods, on a regular basis, are not good for us. As I discussed earlier some of the health consequences of high fat foods are stroke, heart attack and diabetes. It is true that high fat foods usually taste really good but over the long term consuming high fat foods will lead to serious health problems.

Of all the fats available in our foods always try to avoid saturated fat and trans fats. A saturated fat is easy to detect because it will remain solid at room temperature.

Here are some foods that are high in saturated fat:

- Palm oil
- Hydrogenated oils
- Partially hydrogenated oils

If you eat foods with saturated fats you will find it much more difficult to lose weight.

Fat Fact:

Fat contains double the number of calories as the same portion of carbohydrates or protein. Another 'rule of thumb' is that your calories intake should be no more than 30% from fat, any more than that and you will begin to gain weight.

Here are some common high fat foods:

- Doughnuts
- French Fries
- Fried bacon
- Butter
- Pastries
- Mayonnaise
- Olives
- American and Cheddar cheese

As you can see I have included foods that you consider to be 'junk foods' and other foods you would believe to be healthy. Healthy foods will provide a nutritional value to your meals even though there is a fat component within those foods. As I stated earlier, you should limit your fat intake to 30% of your total daily calories so choosing healthy foods that provide the fuel your body needs and are also lower in fat is a crucial component to your weight loss success.

High-Carb Foods

There has been considerable attention given to low-carb diets and how people have had great success losing weight using this type of diet. There is merit to the low carb diet but before you embark on this path let's take a minute to look at how carbohydrates work.

When you consume carbohydrates your body breaks them down into sugar which provides your body with fuel for energy. There are two types of carbohydrates: simple and complex.

What is the difference between a simple and complex carbohydrate? A simple carbohydrate is broken down immediately by your body. This provides a quick source of energy.

The fact that simple carbs are an immediate source of energy is good under the right circumstances however if you load up on simple carbs and are not active then the sugars from the simple carbs are stored as fat. This is where the problem begins, if the sugars are not used for energy they are stored as fat and will not be used by your body until you become more active. If you are not active then the stored fat just accumulates in your body. Our bodies are very intelligent so carbs and calories are used first and stored fats are used later. Again if you are not active the fat keeps piling on.

Like simple carbs complex carbs are broken down and converted into sugar however your body takes longer to break down the complex carbs. The advantage to your body is that by taking longer to break down the complex carbohydrates your body has a more constant and even energy source. This means that the sugars derived from complex carbohydrates do not build up over time like the simple carbohydrates.

It is important for you to include both types of carbohydrates in your diet. Having said that, if you lead a relatively sedentary lifestyle you need to be aware of how your body deals with carbohydrates. Why? Because your sedentary lifestyle will not allow your body to use the energy from the carbs, instead it will all be stored as fat.

Now you can use this information to plan the types of food you use for your meals. If you know you are going to have a relaxed, quiet evening at home plan a dinner that does not include simple carbohydrates and minimizes the amount of complex carbohydrates. No exercise, no movement means your body will not use the energy from the carbs and will store it as fat and that is exactly what we do not want.

I have provided a partial list of simple carbohydrates that we consume almost every day.

Simple Carbohydrates

- Biscuits
- Honey
- Soft drinks
- Chocolate
- Licorice
- Jam

- Cake
- Apples
- Pears
- Raspberries
- Grapefruit
- Cherries

The above list includes 'junk-foods' and healthier simple carbs. The fruits that are listed are simple carbs however they contain simple sugars which means they will not add to your weight problems and they offer many health benefits.

Below you will find a list of common complex carbohydrates.

Complex Carbohydrates

- Brown rice
- Potatoes
- Brown bread
- Bagel
- Corn
- Yams
- Beans
- Peas
- Lentils
- Pasta
- Wholegrain cereals

As I stated earlier complex carbs take a lot longer to break down so they provide your body with a sustained, slow form of energy.

What does this mean to you when you are trying to lose weight? It means you need to closely monitor your intake of carbohydrates and if you are not active then you shouldn't increase the level of carbohydrate intake.

This bears repeating, when you consume carbohydrates your body converts the carbs into sugars and these sugars provide energy for your muscles and body. If you consume carbohydrates and aren't active, the sugars are converted and stored as fat which will be used by your body at a later time. The human body is programmed to burn the most recent energy source first. The consequence is if you are not creating the calorie deficit I talked about earlier then it will be much more difficult to lose weight because of the additional stored fat for the carbohydrates.

So Where Does That Leave Us?

Your nutrition is one of the main tools you use to lose weight. It is imperative that you develop a well-rounded and easy to implement nutritional plan. Being serious about this and making sure you stick with it will make an enormous difference in the amount of weight you will lose. The key is finding the right foods and combine that with the right exercises and when you do this you will reach your weight loss goals.

At this point I need to stress that you can still eat all your favorite foods. However you must be aware of portion size but never starve yourself. Your meals must be filling and satisfying. The mistake you can make is to eat a meal that leaves you unfulfilled and hungry. When you do this you will find that you are craving more food and then your nutritional plan begins to fall apart.

Here are a few suggestions when you are creating your nutritional plan:

- **Make sure you include foods from all four groups**. If you do this you will have a well-rounded and nutritionally sound plan. If you focus on one food group more than the others then your plan will be bland, boring and will destine you to failure. The other consequence is that you will not be supplying your body with all the nutrients it needs to function properly, so take foods from all the groups and enjoy the variety that is available to you.
- **Control your calories.** Don't put a meal together at the last minute and don't keep eating until you are full. In those moments when you are going to eat too much just think of all the work it is going to take to burn off the extra calories.
- **Avoid high fat foods.** These foods will pack on the pounds. You can treat yourself, on occasion, with a piece of cake or a small ice cream, just don't make it a part of every meal.

- **Keep a close eye on carbs.** When you eat carbs make sure that you have a physical activity planned. You need carbs for energy but if you eat a diet heavy in carbs you will put on weight.
- **Drink water and then drink some more water.** Your body needs water, as much water as you can give it because the body uses that water to clear toxins and waste.

To lose weight you need to educate yourself. You need a plan because without a plan you won't know where you are starting and you certainly won't know where you will finish. A concrete, well thought out, practical plan will be a critical component in your long term weight loss success so take the time now and you will thank yourself later.

If you change how you eat you will lose weight but when you incorporate an exercise plan along with the nutritional plan your weight loss will be much more dramatic and long lasting.

Getting Active

Please don't get anxious when you hear you have to exercise. I am not asking you to run a marathon or spend hours in a gym. You need just enough exercise to push you to the 500 calorie deficit and that's all. Common sense goes along way when it comes to exercise.

Without exercise your body can't burn the calories needed to lose weight. Without exercise calories turn into fat and that is what we are trying to avoid.

Exercise: Make It Part Of Your Life

There are those who firmly believe that going to get a snack from the fridge during a commercial qualifies as exercise. I'm sorry to have to tell those people that they are wrong. For an activity to qualify as exercise your heart rate must be raised for a period of time and your muscles must work so that the calories you consumed will be burned off in your muscles.

Some people don't think that a leisurely stroll around the block, or walking up a flight of stairs is exercise. It is exercise and if this is all you can fit into your day then keep doing it. But if you were to sit down and think about exercise what pops into your head, maybe a long walk or playing with your kids? Exercise is any activity which makes you exert yourself.

Why Exercise Is Important

Exercise is fundamental to losing weight. Without exercise your body cannot burn calories but that isn't the only benefit we get from exercise. Here are several benefits of exercise you may not have thought of:

- Exercise gets our hearts pumping and that keeps us healthy. Our heart is a muscle and needs exercise on a regular basis to stay in shape.
- Exercise, when done consistently, has been proven to reduce the stress levels in our bodies. When you exercise your brain releases chemicals that make you feel good and that is a powerful tool to help you reach your goals.
- Exercise is responsible for benefits we are not even aware of such as improving memory, increasing bone density, increased flexibility and a general increase in the quality of your life.
- Exercise has been linked to a longer life so exercise and enjoy every day.
- Exercise strengthens your immune system. Exercise promotes a good night's sleep. It has been proven that sleeping undisturbed through the night is an important key to losing weight.
- Exercise will increase your strength and endurance.

The benefits of exercise are numerous and exercise is an important part of a healthy life. Science and medicine now realize just how important exercise is in keeping us healthy and allowing us to live longer. Take advantage of every opportunity to get out and move, go for a walk, rake your yard, or even do some stretching exercises. When you begin to exercise your body will respond because that is how it has learned to survive for millions of years. Your body wants to work efficiently so give it every opportunity to fulfill its mission, so exercise, eat right, and enjoy life.

Exercise: Do It At Home

You can create an effective exercise plan to do at home and not have to go to a gym. It doesn't have to be a world class exercise workout because our goal is to burn 500 calories more than we consume. That being the case, what should the exercise plan be?

Believe it or not household chores have actually been given a calorie burning value. The following list is based on one hour of activity for a 190 lb. person.

- Working on your car - 259 calories
- Do carpentry work around your home - 302
- Heavy housework (vigorous) - 388
- Light housework - 302
- Laundry - 216
- Preparing meals - 216
- Working in your gardening - 431
- Moving or rearranging furniture - 518
- Yard work – 345

You can see that every day activities provide you with the opportunity to burn calories. Look at it this way, your yard will be immaculate, your house will be spotless, and you will be in great shape!

With the activities listed above you could probably burn off some calories but not enough to make the 500 calorie deficit mark. That means you need to increase your activity level so that you can reach your calorie burning and weight loss goals. It is important that you gradually increase the amount and the intensity of your exercise.

If you haven't done any exercise in years you have to start slow and take the time to let you and your body adjust to the new activities. If you have exercised in the recent past you still need to give your body time to adjust to any increase in your activity level. The worst outcome is that you rush your exercise level and injure yourself. That means you cannot do any activity and you are now in jeopardy of putting on weight while your injury heals.

Before you begin any exercise program be sure to see your personal physician and get their approval and consent.

Here is a list of activities you can do to increase the level of activity. The calorie amounts are based on doing the activity for one hour.

Let's start with light exercise.

- A bike ride - 345
- Stretching - 345
- Yard work - 474
- Jumping rope (slow) - 690
- Shoveling snow - 518
- Treadmill - 518

Light exercise is easy to incorporate into your life and you will see huge benefits from doing light exercise every day.

After you have been doing light exercise and you feel you are in better physical condition you can move onto the following moderate level exercises.

All the following exercises can be done in your home and the calorie numbers are based on one hour of activity.

- Low impact aerobics - 431
- High impact aerobics – 604
- Riding your bike (12-14 mph) – 690
- Riding a stationary bike (moderate effort) – 604
- Golfing and carrying your clubs – 474
- Hiking over moderate terrain – 518
- Jogging – 604
- Jumping rope (moderate) – 863
- Jogging (11 minute mile) – 776
- Rollerblading – 604
- Swimming – 518
- Rowing machine (light effort) – 819

- Basketball – 388
- Push-ups and sit-ups - 690

One of the best casual activities is probably a brisk walk.

You can burn 345 calories if you take a longer walk.

You should not attempt these exercises without the permission of your physician.

To take your exercise to the next level here are the heavy exercises. These exercises will get your heart pumping, your calorie burning through the roof and the pounds dropping off.

Many of the activities are the same as the light and medium exercises but you just use a higher energy level.

- Biking (16-19 mph steady pace for one hour). You burn over 1000 calories for every hour you ride your bike at a good speed.
- Canoeing (over 6 mph) - 1035
- Running (6 minute mile) - 1380
- Ice hockey - 690
- Jumping rope (fast) - 1035
- Cross-country skiing - between 600 and 1400 calories depending on effort
- Squash - 1035
- Swimming (from treading water to the butterfly stroke) - 500 to 950

Finding An Exercise Program That Is Right For You

This is where your lifestyle can collide with your new plan. You are so busy that you might find it difficult to find one hour of free time to exercise. The hard cold fact is that you will not be able to lose weight unless you are able to exercise. You must make the commitment to set aside the time and provide yourself with the opportunity to reach all your weight loss goals.

Keep in mind that you don't have to exercise to the point where you are gasping for breath, but the more intense the exertion the more calories you burn and the faster you reach your goals. Everything you do during your day counts as calorie burning activity. If you do these activities with a little more exertion and use more energy you will get closer and closer to your 500 calories deficit goal.

Here are a couple of suggestions to help you find the time to exercise every day.

- Walk past the elevator and take the stairs. It will not be easy but after you do this for a week or two it will get easier. You will feel great and you will know you are burning those calories. You might even get to the point where you walk past your floor and then come back down, and then you know you have made enormous progress.
- This one is definitely difficult but not for the reasons you think. Here it is, get up one hour earlier and go for a long brisk walk. Because you got up earlier you will eat earlier. This means that your metabolism gets the fuel it needs and you are ready to burn calories. Just think, it is still early in the day and you are on your way to reach your calorie deficit goals.
- When you do housework, scrub a little harder and vacuum a little quicker. Try walking faster when you mow the lawn. Everything counts and everything adds up.
- Join a local sport club. Try basketball, or go to aerobics, try to find an activity you can do for several hours over the course of the week. If you do this you are heading straight to the winners circle for weight loss.
- This might be too expensive, but buy or rent a piece of home exercise equipment. If you buy it make sure you use it, you won't lose any weight just watching the equipment gather dust. If you enjoy reading at night then get on your treadmill and read while you walk.

Remember that any exercise helps you reach your goals. Find the time in your schedule and try to exercise three times a week. Regular exercise will get you to your weight loss goals quicker.

The benefits of regular exercise go beyond losing weight. Anyone who had a sedentary lifestyle must begin to move and work up to an exercise routine. It is a matter of life or death.

What Are Your Diets Plan Options?

You probably have been overwhelmed by the number of diet plans that promise "Lose 10lbs. in 10 days'. These plans do not offer you a plan you can use for the rest of your life. What they offer is a quick fix that will get the weight off but if you use those plans the weight will come roaring back as soon as you stop the diet. That doesn't mean that all diet plans are bad it just means that some make promises that are unreasonable and not life changing.

I am sure you are familiar with all the 'Big' names in the diet world, plans like Jenny Craig, Weight Watchers, NutriSystem and so many more. I bet you have been thinking that somewhere out there is the diet plan for you. Well, in this section I will be discussing the different diet plans and at the very end I will tell you what my plan is. So let's get going.

The Plans

From my research I believe that there are approximately six diet plan options that give you a reasonable weight loss plan. Each plan has its own particular strengths and weaknesses but they all offer you a decent plan. .As you are probably aware, some of these plans require you to join a club and buy pre-packaged foods steering you away from the foods they consider 'bad' and buy only the foods they believe are 'good'.

It would take too long to go into every detail of each program so instead I will give you an overview of the programs and a short list of what I believe are the 'Pros' and 'Cons' of each plan. My goal is to present important information you can use to make fundamental changes in your life.

The Atkins Diet

This diet has been in the news for a few years. It is a low-carb diet and that is the primary method this diet uses to reduce weight. The other important feature of this plan is that you consume high protein foods such as meat, eggs, and seafood as well as monounsaturated fats, i.e., cheeses, butter, sausages, etc.

When you first begin the Atkins Diet you are in what is called the 'induction phase.' What does that mean? It means that in the first two weeks of starting the

Atkins Diet you cannot eat more than 20 grams of carbohydrates per day. These carbohydrates are usually derived from vegetables but you have to avoid high carbohydrate foods such as potatoes, carrots and corn.

The way the Atkins diet works is that you can increase your carbohydrates by 5 grams every week until you hit a predetermined maximum (total) of between 40 to 90 grams. When you reach that point in the Atkins diet you are considered to be in the 'maintenance' phase.

Here are the Pros and Cons as I see them:

Pros

- You lose weight on the Atkins Diet. Millions of people will attest to that.
- Your carbohydrate intake is very controlled and to a certain degree that is good.
- The Atkins Diet endorses that a dieter must put a limit on the number of high sugar and processed foods they consume.

Cons

- The most recent scientific research endorses eating more fruits and vegetables. On the Atkins Diet the consumption of these food groups is limited.
- High fat foods such as red meat, which is a fundamental food group in the Atkins, cause problems for our hearts and might be linked to serious illnesses.
- We use protein to build muscle but on the Atkins Diet there are few carbohydrates to burn for energy. It is true that consuming protein will lead to weight loss but without the carbohydrates in the diet your body may resort to using your lean muscle mass for energy. That is never good.
- Only small portions of carbohydrates are allowed on a weekly basis, 40 to 90 grams, and this goes against everything modern science and nutrition believes is healthy.

The conclusion is that with the Atkins Diet you will lose weight however due to the structure of the diet, high fat and low carb, it may not be a healthy diet over the long run. Remember, we are looking for a diet plan that we can use for the rest of our lives not just for a few months.

A study was done on people using the Atkins diet. The study found that up to 40% stopped using the Atkins Diet plan within 12 months. The people stated that the diet was just too hard to stay on. However the remaining 60% did lose weight, an average of 16 lbs. in the first six months. But the weight loss dropped to 10 lbs. after one year on the Atkins Diet.

One of the fundamental reasons people stop a diet is that they miss all the foods they had to give up and this is one of the reasons people find the Atkins Diet difficult to use for an extended period of time.

As discussed earlier, our bodies are very intelligent. If our body detect that something is missing, it will send us a message which we call a 'craving'. As soon as you stop a diet that restricted your foods you will begin eating the foods you craved and as you do you will gain all the weight back.

Low Carb Diets

Our bodies do not know the difference between a spoonful of sugar or a bite from an apple. To our bodies it doesn't matter because it all gets converted into sugar. Our bodies have to have sugar for fuel and without sugar we are in trouble.

A low-carb diet is based on limiting our carbohydrate intake. This results in our body experiencing times when there are no carbs to burn and when our body faces that situation it will burn fat. A low carb diet is similar to Atkins however it does not go as far as Atkins in limiting carbohydrate consumption.

The basic principle behind a low carb diet is to create a shortage or deficiency of sugar in our body. This shortage of sugar forces our bodies to burn fat and if you burn fat you lose weight.

A low carb diet differs from the Atkins diet in that the low carb diet will limit you to the lower end of the recommended daily intake of carbs. A low carb diet also requires you to reduce or completely stop consuming the quick simple sugars that are in foods.

Remember, simple carbohydrates are broken down quickly which allows the sugars to immediately enter your blood supply. On the other hand the body takes longer to break down complex carbohydrates and this longer breakdown time provides your body with a sustained energy source. The problem begins when you consume large amounts of simple carbs and then do not have any physical activity. The sugars are then converted immediately to fat. When you consume simple sugars you must accompany that with some type of physical activity.

Pros

- You will consume less simple carbs. This means two things - first, you will limit the amount of sugars that your body has to burn immediately, and second because you are limiting your simple carbs you are not consuming all the fat that goes along with this food group (not fruits and some vegetables). Remember, you are on a diet so you are trying to reduce the amount of fat you consume.
- With a reasonable level of physical activity you will burn the small amount of sugar that you are consuming and then you will begin to burn fat. This is what we want!
- You can consume some of the carbs you like but not at the same level as Atkins.

Cons

- Weight loss will occur, however you will have to give up many of the foods you like, just like in the Atkins Diet. This might become a problem in keeping the weight off for the long term.
- A strict adherence to this diet might mean that you go too far in reducing your carbohydrates and too severely limit yourself from healthy fruits, vegetables, beans, legumes and whole grains.

It is a good idea to reduce the carbs in your diet as long as you aren't reducing to the point of limiting the important fruits and vegetables and missing out on important nutrients.

To be successful in a low carb diet you must like foods low in carbohydrates. I realize that saying that sound painfully obvious but people do not always think about the implications of a diet. To be successful on a low carbohydrate diet you have to enjoy eating meats, cheeses, poultry and other high protein foods. These are the types of foods a low carb diet is based on.

Low Fat Diet

This is probably the most popular diet. This is so popular because you can still eat many of your favorite foods you just can't eat them all the time.

The reason why these diets are so popular is because it is common knowledge that fat = calories.   This is absolutely true; fat is the most dense food we eat in terms of calories. So it just makes sense that the less fat we eat the fewer calories we consume which will in turn make it easier for you to lose weight. However there is something you must be aware of. It is not healthy to remove all fat from your diet. There are two kinds of fat and you need to know the differences. The first group of fats I will call the 'Bad' Fats.

Bad Fats

Bad fats are saturated and trans-fats. I spoke about these fats earlier but did not explain why we consider then 'bad'. These fats are 'bad' or unhealthy for us to eat because they are linked to cardiovascular disease. Another reason these fats are bad for us is that they raise our cholesterol more than any other food item in our diet.

If your diet consists of foods that raise your cholesterol then the following will happen: your arteries begin to get clogged which makes them smaller and restricts the flow of blood through your body. As a result of your arteries being clogged your heart has to work much harder to pump the blood through all your arteries. If your arteries become so clogged that the blood cannot circulate then you have reached a point of having a life changing event, a very bad event.

The fat that is considered the worst of the bad fats is trans-fat. Another method to identify a fat as a trans-fat is if you see partially hydrogenated on the label. It is almost guaranteed that the product contains trans-fats. Trans-fats lower the good cholesterol (HDL) and raise the bad cholesterol (LDL).The only purpose of trans-fats is to increase the shelf life of the food item; there is no nutritional value to a trans-fat.

Good Fats

Good fats are monounsaturated and polyunsaturated fats. These types of fats contain elements that aid proper cell structure, the production of hormones and these fats get stored for energy.

Monounsaturated and polyunsaturated fats contain Omega-3 fatty acids, which have been shown to reduce heart disease, diabetes, stroke, and high blood pressure. It is difficult to see how you could go wrong consuming something that reduces the chances of getting those terrible diseases. Anytime you can consume something that reduces those devastating diseases, you are doing exactly what you should be doing.

Pros

- Low Fat diets are one of the easiest methods to lose weight. By reducing the level of fats in your diet you also limit your calories. Think of how this would help you reach your 500 calories daily deficit.
- Your favorite foods are still on your menu. You won't find yourself craving your favorites and although the foods you eat might be high in carbs it is also low in fat and that's the key to this diet.
- You can eat from all food groups. Take your pick, carbs, fat, proteins and nutrients are all part of and important to this diet.

Cons

- If you go overboard and cut out all fats, you might be losing some very important fats that will help in developing healthy cells and storing energy.
- This diet makes it easy to cheat. It is very easy to grab a piece of cake, a chocolate bar, or other favorite when you don't have a restrictive diet. If in your mind fat doesn't equal calories then you might not be able to sustain this diet.
- As with any diet you have to be committed to making the diet work. This might mean not being able to eat all of your favorite foods. So commitment

is absolutely critical. Take a look at the diet and then be honest with yourself and decide whether you can commit to this program.

Weight Watchers / Jenny Craig

Weight Watchers and Jenny Craig are two of the most popular diet plans. They are both advertised very heavily on TV and other media. One of the main concepts behind each of these plans is counting calories. Both Weight Watchers and Jenny Craig have their own line of foods and supplements that are high in protein but low in sugars and fats. With Jenny Craig you purchase the meals directly from them as opposed to Weight Watchers where you purchase their food at the supermarket.

A strong point of both plans is the support from other members and it probably is no surprise that the support is a strong selling point. It is proven that people who have a support system stand a much greater chance of succeeding at weight loss because everyone enjoys having people cheer them on and help them over the hurdles.

These two benefits, the support and the food, make Weight Watchers and Jenny Craig two of the most popular plans available today.

Pros

- You don't have to think about preparing meals. The prepared meals make the decision of what to eat pretty easy.
- These plans have been available for quite a few years so they have a proven track record.
- Support. There is no question that having a support system will increase your chances of being successful at weight loss.

Cons

- You have to pay for the prepackaged meals. You can save money making your own meals.
- What happens when you get tired of the plan? It is possible with these plans that you do not take full responsibility for your food intake. If you tire of these plans what will you do to keep the weight off?

Diet Pills

Diet pills are a controversial subject. Some people swear by them and others believe that no one should ever take a diet pill. There is growing evidence that diet pills can be harmful but for someone who is desperate to lose weight diet pills may seem like a viable option.

There have been studies that have examined the long-term risks and effects of taking diet pills. As of now the studies seem to indicate that there might be some obese-related diseases that are curbed by using diet pills. The research indicates that diet pills might:

- Lower blood pressure
- Decrease insulin resistance
- Lower cholesterol

But the long-term studies are not conclusive. Diet pills are intended to help someone on a diet stay on the diet by suppressing the urge to eat but many people take diet pills and believe that the pills are a 'cure' for being overweight. Before you take diet pills, be aware that these pills do present a risk.

Pros

- You will lose weight.

- You don't have to change what you eat to lose weight.

Cons

- The possibility that the person taking the pills will become dependent on the pills. Most of the commercially available diet pills are particularly habit forming but the effect these pills have on a person's appetite can be addictive.
- There have not been enough studies to determine if there are long term side effects to diet pills. If you take these pills prior to knowing exactly what these pills do to you long term, then you are putting yourself at risk.
- Diet pills give people a false sense of what is possible when they are losing weight. Diet pills allow a person to lose weight fast however what happens when the person no longer takes the pills.

- As with any drug your body can build up a tolerance to that drug over time. It has been shown that diet pills will not be as effective after 5 - 6 months of use. People find that their weight loss slows down and levels off at that time.

All of the plans I have spoken about have strengths and weaknesses and each will help you lose weight. The most difficult aspect of any diet is sticking to it over the long term.

Important! You should ALWAYS consult your physician if you are think diet pills are a viable option for your diet plan. Also you should consult your doctor about any weight loss program you want to begin.

You need to make a commitment to nutrition and exercise in order to make your fight against your beltline a successful one. No diet or support group will take the weight off for you. To be successful you must make the commitment to changing your life.

My Weight Loss Plan

I'm not going to give you a specific list of foods or the exact exercise routines to do every day. What I am going to do is change the way you view food and exercise so that you can be in control of all aspects of the weight loss process. This is your life so you need to know what works for you and when changes need to be made you will need the information to make intelligent and insightful decisions.

As you know I have talked from the very beginning about the 500 calories daily deficit. That mean you will have to commit to eating 250 less calories and burning 250 more calories every day. When you do this you will lose 1lb. every week. Each day you will be getting closer to your goal and in two months you will have lose 8 lbs.

It is possible to lose more weight if you want. All you need to do is increase the level of your daily calorie deficit and then adjust how many calories you eat and how many calories you need to burn. How you do that is entirely up to you. But, I do have some suggestions you might want to follow so you will be confident you are consuming the correct number of calories.

(1) Reduce the fat content in your diet. By doing this you will lower your caloric intake.

(2) Be very aware of your portion sizes. Make sure your portion sizes are smaller and that you eat slower and chewing your food well. Doing this will bring you two benefits, first, by eating smaller portions and eating slower you will actually feel full quicker. Also, when you put together smaller portions with slower eating you get one thing - less calories.

(3) Exercise at least three days out of the week. This is the minimum you can do and lose weight. If you manage to incorporate physical activity five day a week you will accelerate your weight loss and make dramatic changes in your metabolism.

(4) Always make sure you eat a balanced diet. You must include foods from all four food groups if you are serious about creating a healthy, well balanced nutritional plan.

(5) Remember that empty calories are your enemy. This might sound like a cliché, but it is the truth. Junk food or fast food provides you with a heavy load of empty calories and simple carbohydrates. You now know what overloading on simple carbs means, it means you are packing on fat.

Exercise

Exercise is essential to losing weight. If you are serious about and truly committed to losing weight then you have no alternative but to increase your activity level. Without exercise you will never be able to create your daily calorie deficit and without that you will not lose weight.

Don't limit your thinking when it comes to exercise. Exercise is any physical activity that raises your heart rate and keeps it elevated for at least 20 minutes. If you have the time to go to a gym then go, but if you do not have the time then be creative in how you achieve your weight loss exercise. Exercise = calories burned and that plus your reduced portion sizes and low fat meals means you will be losing all the weight you want.

Here are a few suggestions regarding exercise:

- Start slow and build up. When you get to a comfortable level and feel you are doing everything you can add 10% more exercise to your exercise routine.
- Don't create obstacles in your mind about exercise. You are not expected to be a world class athlete. You are expected to do everything you can to reach your weight loss goals so find as many ways possible to add activity and exercise into your day. Set your goal to burn 250 calories and work up from there.
- Get the approval of your primary care physician before you get involved in a strenuous sport. If you rush into an activity that is too strenuous and makes demands on your body that it is not prepared for, you could injure yourself. Depending on the injury you could set yourself back for weeks.
- You have to burn calories so find something that you enjoy doing and then the burning of calories won't seem like work.
- Activities are always more enjoyable when you can share them with others. Try to enlist a friend or family member to exercise with you. When you have support and you are having fun then there is a much greater probability you will continue with the activity.
- Losing weight is a lifestyle change and exercise is part of that change. Make this a true lifestyle change and not a change just to lose weight.

Nutrition

I have talked about all the different diet plans, the different types of fat, cholesterol, carbohydrates and more. It really boils down to a very simple concept: how many calories you eat during the day and how many of those calories you burn off during the day.

To give yourself the best chance of being successful, just control your calories. When you are successful at controlling your calories then you will be losing weight.

Here is a brief outline:

- Find your target body mass index or your target weight.

- Determine the number of calories you need to maintain that weight. This is where you find your 500 calorie deficit.
- Eat the foods you need to stay at or below your target calorie consumption. Remember to work into your nutritional plan your vitamins and minerals.
- Never skip a meal to reach your calorie intake level. Skipping a meal will adversely affect your metabolism and that is the last thing you want to do. If you missed your calories goal by 100 calories just work a little longer in your exercise time and burn them off. Just don't make a habit of missing your goals.
- Avoid saturated or trans-fats. These are the worst kinds of fats. These fats clog your arteries and make your heart work harder just to get the blood through your body.

Your diet and your exercise, coupled together, will determine how successful you will be in reaching your weight loss goals. You must eat a healthy, well balanced diet and although this might not be as flashy as a fad diet, a well-balanced nutritional plan coupled with exercise will over the long haul allow you to reach your long term weight loss goals. Don't rely on the quick fix of diet pills, you may lose weight but you have nothing to fall back on after the pills stop working.

Words of Wisdom:

To achieve long term weight loss, never equate the weight loss program you have chosen with a diet. It is so much more than just reducing calories, it is a life style change that you will have for the rest of your life.

Getting A Plan Set Up

I've given you pages and pages of information regarding how to establish a diet plan that will work for you. As the above 'Words of Wisdom' say, don't think of your weight loss journey as just a diet, always remember that this is a life style change. You understand that controlling your weight is now a top priority for and you also know that you will have to make many changes in addition to just your eating to be successful.

You are now mentally ready to begin the discovery of the new you by establishing your weight loss plan. There will be some days when everything works fine, you eat everything you should, you exercise and your thinking is pushing you forward. There will also be days when nothing works, your eating is outside your plan, you didn't exercise and your thinking is not focused on success. This is going to happen no matter who you are so do not let a day like this derail your long term weight loss goals. Take the day for what it is, just one day in your life. A 'bad' day isn't the end of the world if you see it for what it is. At the end of the day tell yourself that you are going to get back on track as soon as you wake up and then get a good night's rest. Tomorrow is a new day filled with opportunities for success, contentment, and progress. When you are ready for the inevitable 'ups and downs' of this journey you will be able to ride them out and stay on course.

I touched on this earlier, but here is a list of things you can do to make your weight loss journey successful.

- Set realistic weight loss goals. If your goal is to lose 10 pounds, 30 pounds or 100 pounds, then go for it. It is very important to have specific and achievable weight loss goals. Make sure that you have your 'big' goal of the total number of pounds you are going to lose and make sure that you have smaller goals. Goals you reach in one week that will keep you moving forward and building momentum to achieve you next goal.
- There will be some changes, some people may think of them as challenges that you will have to adjust to. Be willing to make these changes and meet these challenges. When you hit a 'roadblock' think of it in terms of helping you because as you overcome the roadblock you will be stronger, wiser, more determined, and closer to your goal. How you perceive and react to every situation you encounter on your weight loss journey will have an enormous effect on your success.
- Sacrifices, there will be times when you will have to sacrifice something. Maybe it is exercising instead of watching TV, or passing up your favorite dessert even though you have stuck to all your nutritional plans that day. Whatever form the sacrifice takes be willing and ready to move past it. It is only a sacrifice if you think of your weight loss as less important than what has your attention at the moment.
- Determine your body mass index and your ideal weight then determine how you will reach your ideal weight.

- Determine you caloric intake to reach and maintain your ideal weight. Now you know how many calories you need each day to create your 500 calorie daily deficit.
- Take a few minutes to think about and write down a typical day's meals and the number of calories you will consume in that day. Be honest because if you cheat you are only deceiving and hurting yourself.
- Once you know how many calories you will consume on a typical day then plan out your exercise so you can burn up at least 250 calories each day.
- You are now at the point where you can begin making adjustments to your meal plans and exercise to cut even more calories. You need to determine how you can reduce calories from your diet. It really is as straight forward as that. You can reduce calories by eating smaller portions, not having any dessert or pass on the chips or soda at lunch.

Now look at your exercise, where can you increase your activity level? Can you take a walk after work, spend 15 minutes more on the treadmill, or play with the kids for a few more minutes after dinner? Be creative and find as many ways as you can to increase your activity level.

- Write your plan down and stick with it. In the beginning it will feel strange but soon it will feel completely natural. Attack your plan with unswerving dedication and enthusiasm. Don't get discouraged in the beginning; you are in this for the long haul.
- In 30 days re-evaluate your plan, how is it working, what changes need to be made, how can you improve your meals and exercise? As soon as you begin to feel bored or your meals seem unsatisfying sit down and evaluate the plan. Believe in yourself and your ability to make the changes you need to make to reach your weight loss goals.

Above all else, stick with it. Never quit, never doubt yourself, set your goals, take responsibility for your nutrition and exercise, and take responsibility for your success.

You are already on your way to reaching your goals, close your eyes and see yourself one year from today. Now that you overcame all the obstacles, all the sacrifices, and all the exercise and there you stand having lost all that weight, how do you feel? You are already there just follow your vision and you will succeed. You have embarked on a course that will change you forever.

Conclusion

Congratulations! You have taken the action to change your life. You have committed to losing weight and making all the lifestyle changes required. I have given you as much information as I can and hopefully you reinforced this information so you have the tools, the mindset, and the focus to attack your weight loss and reach all your goals.

Just think of where you will be in one year, you will have lost a lot of weight and you will have begun and maintained a healthier lifestyle. The changes you made have lowered your risk for heart disease, stroke, high blood pressure and many other illnesses.

In just a few months you will be able to do things you were not able to do before embarking on this journey. You will be fitter and lighter. You are now in control of your food, your exercise, your life, and your weight.

The entire world is waiting for you to explore and enjoy. All that is standing in your way is your weight but now you know how to lose that weight and live a new, fuller life.

I wish you a life filled with joy and contentment!

Kelley O'Hara

Website Resources With Great Information

The Internet has been a tremendous revolution for the flow of information. You can research almost anything in the world on the Internet. Losing weight and keeping it off are no different.

There are vast resources and information on dieting and losing weight, and in many cases it is probably best to be as informed as possible about what you are getting into before you take the time to do it. But, if you are looking for information the Internet is the place to get it. There will be times when just the sheer amount of information will be overwhelming or confusing and when you find yourself in that position consult your personal physician.

I have put together a few of the websites I found to be very useful. You can benefit from the information and it will only take a few minutes to view each site. These are in no particular order, and I have included comments on each site.

http://www.freedieting.com/tools/calorie_calculator.htm

This is where you can find a caloric needs calculator that will assist you in finding the information to maintain your weight and help you find ways to reach the 500 calorie daily deficit.

http://www.nutristrategy.com/activitylist4.htm

This site provides general information for many daily exercises and activities. This information will assist you in determining how much energy you are expending during your average day, and how much exercise you need to add to that to burn off the calories.

http://www.thecolumn.org/dieting-tips.asp

This site contains information and tips that you can put to use right away. You will find information on dieting and a dieting forum.

http://www.americanheart.org/presenter.jhtml?identifier=1480

This is one of the best sites for getting information on losing weight. Everyone knows that your heart is affected by how overweight or obese you are. This site will give you tips and information that will help you now and over the months.

http://www.free-weight-loss-resources.com/

This site is filled with 'free' resources on fitness and dieting.

http://www.halls.md/ideal-weight/body.htm

This site will provide you with some insight to your weight and where your target weight should be.

http://www.cfsan.fda.gov/~dms/wh-wght.html

This site is a government site and has a lot of information on many aspects of weight loss and the effects of obesity.